How To Fight Osteoporosis and Win!

The Miracle of Microcrystalline Hydroxyapatite (MCHC)

A Health Learning Handbook
By Beth M. Ley

BL Publications, Aliso Viejo, CA 92656, (714) 452-0371

Library of Congress Cataloging- In Publication Data

Ley, Beth M. 1964-
    How to Fight Osteoporosis and Win! The Miracle of Microcrystalline Hydroxyapatite (MCHC) / by Beth M. Ley. -- 1st Ed.
            p.   cm.
Includes biographical references and index
ISBN 0-9642703-5-8 (alk. paper)
    1. Osteoporosis--Popular works.
    2. Osteoporosis--Chemotherapy.
3. Hydroxyapatite--Therapeutic use.   I. Title.
RC931.073L49 1996
616.7'16--dc20   96-27467
                                                  CIP

ISBN: 0-9642703-5-8

Printed in the United States of America

First edition, August 1996.

How to Fight Osteoporosis and Win: The Miracle of Microcrystalline Hydroxyapatite is not intended as medical advice. Its intention is solely informational and educational. It is wise to consult your doctor for any illness or medical condition. This publication may not be distributed through mail order companies without the written approval of BL Publications.

Credits:
Typesetting and Cover Design: BL Publications
Editing: Victoria Earhart, Kim DeLaura, Roslyn Schryver

TABLE OF CONTENTS

Introduction

Health Learning Handbooks are designed to provide useful information about ways to improve one's health and well-being. Education about what the body needs to obtain and maintain good health is what we would like to provide.

Good health should not be thought of as absence of disease. We should avoid negative disease oriented thinking and concentrate on what we have to do to remain healthy. Health is maintaining on a daily basis what is essential to the body. Disease is the result of attempting to live without what the body needs. We are responsible for our own health and should take control of it. If we are in control of our health, disease will not take control.

Our health depends on education.

Bone loss, known as osteoporosis, is a problem so widespread in America today that many authorities refer to it as an epidemic. As bone structure deteriorates faster than it is regenerated, it becomes weak, brittle and fragile.

More than 1.5 million Americans have fractures related to osteoporosis at an annual cost in the U.S. health care system of 10 billion dollars. Complications of hip fractures are a major killer of women. In many cases, the fracture precedes a fall rather than being caused by it. Soft, spongy bone...found in the jaw, hips, spine, and wrists...is the first to go.

Men also, lose bone as the years progress, although only about half as quickly as women.

Great pain is experienced but fortunately osteoporosis is preventable and can be aided with the help of special supplements available over the counter.

In this book you will find out if you are at increased risk for excessive bone loss.

Most importantly you will read about ways to prevent and treat this devastating problem. Prevention is the most economical way to approach this, and almost all other health problems.

In this book, you will learn about the **known** facts of calcium, dairy products, calcium supplements and the health of your bones. This publication is not sponsored by the dairy industry, the pharmaceutical industry or anyone else trying to sell you something, so you can make a decision based on the facts, not on a marketing strategy.

For more information about osteoporosis...

Calcium Information Center :
Calcium Information Line: (toll free) 1-800-321-2681

National Osteoporosis Foundation:
PO Box 96616 Department MQ, Washington, D,C, 20077

Osteoporosis

Osteoporosis is the result of a loss of normal bone density, marked by thinning of bone tissue and the growth of small holes in the bone. Osteoporosis means "porous bone".

Weakened, less dense bones are more susceptible to fractures and breakage. X-rays of osteoporotic bones reveal many hairline fractures in areas such as the lumbar region of the spine. Others areas where hairline fractures are commonly seen are wrist, forearm, leg, and hip. These fractures are not only painful, they further weaken the bone.

Bone cells, like all cells in the body, are continually renewing themselves. This process involves bone reabsorption where minerals are removed from the bones, and bone formation where minerals are put

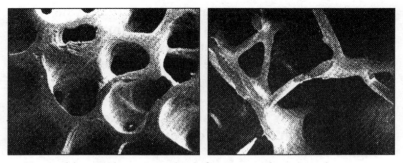

Normal bone shown on the left is more dense and stronger compared to the "thinned" out, porous bone with osteoporosis on the right. This bone is much weaker and more likely to break or fracture.

back into new bone. When bone reabsorption occurs at a faster rate than new bone is formed, the result is bone loss, medically termed *osteoporosis.*

After our third decade, the level of our bone mass plateaus. Bone loss begins in the fourth or fifth decade of life. In women bone loss accelerates after menopause. Among men it accelerates after age 65.

Are you at risk?

Osteoporosis is not inevitable for everyone, but there are numerous factors which increase one's susceptibility to the problem.

Women are more likely to develop osteoporosis than men because men start with a larger bone mass and do not go through the dramatic hormonal changes that women do.

Thin people are more prone to osteoporosis than heavy individuals.

Blacks experience osteoporosis less often than **caucasians** as their bones are generally more dense to begin with.

Women with northern **European** blood ties are of an even higher risk.

Individuals at additional risk are those who take steroid hormones such as **anti-inflammatory agents** commonly prescribed for arthritis and joint discomfort.

Smokers, and those who consume **alcohol** or **caffeine** through coffee. tea, cola, etc., are at a higher risk.

Individuals who consume a diet high in **animal protein** which induces a calcium deficiency, are at a higher risk.

Individuals who consume a large amount of **sweets** and **refined carbohydrates** are at a higher risk.

Individuals who experience prolonged **stress,** or live a **sedentary** life and do not get adequate exercise are at a higher risk.

Secondary osteoporosis is caused as a result of the imbalance caused by another health problem. These include:

Endocrine disorders (such as thyrotoxicosis, Cushing's Syndrome, hypogonadism, hyperparathyroidism, juvenile diabetes mellitus),

Collagen disturbances (such as scurvy, osteogenesis),

Blood disorders (such as sickle cell anemia),

Several types of **Cancer** (myeloma, leukemia and lymphoma).

Other health problems include:

Rheumatoid arthritis,
Chronic renal disease,
Intestinal malabsorption,
Gastrectomy,
Alcoholism and related liver disease.

Symptoms of Osteoporosis

Osteoporosis may be very painful (especially in the lower back), may cause frequent broken bones, loss of body height, and deformities.

Loss of height
Cramps in legs and feet (often at night)
Bone pain
Lower back pain
Fractures of the hip, wrist, spine
Dowager's hump - forward bending of the spine
Fatigue
Brittle or soft fingernails
Premature grey hair
Heart palpitations

Osteoporosis Facts

● During a lifetime women lose approximately 50% of the cancellous bone and 30% of corticol bone. Men lose about 30% and 20% of the same.

● The average American loses 1.5 inches of height <u>each decade</u> after menopause as a result of vertebral collapse. This means you may be 3 inches shorter at 70 than you were at age 50!

● Osteoporosis is the cause of 90 percent of all fractures after age 65.

● One out of every three women over 65 will suffer hip fracture, a catastrophe which is fatal in one out of every five cases.

● Osteoporosis causes 40% of all people to lose their teeth after age 60. (Periodontal disease is osteoporosis of the mouth.)

● Osteoporosis is primarily a disease of "modernized" countries. Not all areas of the world have seen the dramatic increase in the incidence of osteoporosis that we have in the U.S. This may be due to "estrogen dominance" created due to the abundant use of hormones and chemicals in our foods.

● **Men are not exempt.** Most of us think of osteoporosis as a woman's problem. Men are not excluded from this epidemic, statistics show that one out of every six men over 90 will fracture a hip.

● Prevention is by far the easiest and most cost effective approach to osteoporosis.

What Causes Osteoporosis?

One would think that we would have a better handle on the cause of a health problem that affects so many people in such a devastating manner. The truth is that there is no simple answer. There are a combination of factors which lead to bone loss. Some of these we have control over. Some we do not.

Homeostasis

An upset in body chemistry results in increased susceptibility to health problems. When all the minerals, hormones, pH level and other elements are in balance, the body is in homeostasis and the body runs most efficiently. When an imbalance occurs, the body will make certain adjustments with its numerous built-in mechanisms, designed to keep the internal body chemistry in balance.

Changes in the acid base balance of the body is a tremendous contributor to bone loss. Even a slight decrease in pH (increased acidosis) leads to the loss of calcium from bone as the calcium (in the form of calcium chloride, calcium carbonate, or calcium phosphate) is needed as an alkaline buffer. The many causes of increased acidosis are discussed in detail later.

The body functions best when all the needed

nutrients, including minerals, are present in their proper proportions. But if there is a shortage of just one mineral, the system will weaken and begin to lose efficiency. With the balance of the body off, the body cannot operate optimally and eventually disease will set in. In this case, osteoporosis.

Many people assume that osteoporosis is the result of a calcium deficiency. While this may be true in many situations, it is by by no means the only cause of osteoporosis. A better description would perhaps be mineral **imbalance**, but again there are many, many other contributing factors. If other factors are causing a calcium deficiency or what appears to be a calcium deficiency, resulting in the depletion of bone, then the true cause of osteoporosis is **not** a calcium deficiency, but the other factors.

Mineral Balancing

Obtaining enough minerals through the diet is only half of the battle. The other half is maintaining balanced levels among each of the minerals. Dr. Paul Eck, scientist and mineral researcher, probably recognized as one of the foremost authorities in the world on the role of minerals in human health, stresses that mineral imbalances are the underlying cause of most of our health troubles.

For example, according to Dr. Eck, the four main minerals in the body, calcium, magnesium, sodium, and potassium, regulate two areas of critical importance in the body, the thyroid and adrenal glands. If these four minerals are at normal levels, and everything else is in balance, these glands can function optimally.

Imbalances will cause either overactivity which can result in stress or underactivity which results in low energy levels and insufficiency. Calcium and potassium are the two major minerals involved in the activity of the thyroid gland. If the ratio between them and the mineral levels is normal, the thyroid functions at maximum energy levels.

Calcium slows down the activity of the thyroid, and potassium speeds it up. If the level of calcium is too high, the energy level of the thyroid will be slowed down. If the level of potassium is too high, the thyroid will be overactive and will eventually wear out completely because of too much stress.

If one mineral level is too high or too low, it affects all other minerals in the body. No mineral works alone. For example, frequently individuals take an iron supplement because they are tired. This is what can happen: Iron causes sodium levels to rise as a result of stimulating the adrenal glands. Magnesium levels will go down because sodium lowers magnesium. Calcium will go down because magnesium and calcium strive to be at the same level. Calcium and potassium move in opposite directions, so when calcium goes down, potassium goes up. It doesn't end here, since as many as 21 minerals can be affected by altering just one. Again, no mineral works alone.

Calcium

Contrary to popular belief, osteoporosis is not due to a lack of dietary calcium. It is the result of the loss of calcium caused by a number of factors.

The Recommended Daily Requirement (RDA) for calcium for healthy men and women is between 600 and 800 mg. This is not difficult to reach, as you can see by looking over the list of popular foods containing calcium on page 34. The actual amount of calcium an individual needs actually varies. Calcium needs increase with age. Women who have passed menopause need at least 1,500 mg daily. Calcium absorption diminishes as we grow older due to a number of reasons including hormonal and digestive. Vegetarians who tend to consume a "less acidic" diet do not require as much calcium as meat eaters. High protein foods are acid-forming which requires the body to neutralize the low pH. The body does this with calcium.

Calcium deficiencies do occur but it is not known for certain whether deficiencies are due entirely to inadequate intake, or a combination of factors which cause diminished absorption and utilization of the calcium we consume in our foods. Imbalances may be created from a variety of factors. I suspect it often is a combination of all of these things. This theory suggests that supplementation of calcium alone would not solve the problem. And this we know to be true. Simply supplementing calcium **WILL NOT** solve the problem of osteoporosis,

As calcium is very important to our overall health, the body will attempt to regulate calcium levels in the blood, even if this means sacrificing bone. Because of this, laboratory blood tests will usually indicate that calcium and phosphorus levels are normal.

Other Calcium Related Health Problems

Osteoarthritis is a form of arthritis in which one or more joints have abnormal tissue changes. Cartilage which normally cushions the joints becomes soft and breaks down. Small pieces of bone may become loose and get caught inside the joint causing painful bony spikes. Large calcium deposits can make movement very difficult causing a crippling effect.

Mineral imbalances and excess calcium circulating in the blood are thought to be partially responsible for this painful degenerative condition.

The Calcium Regulators: The Parathyroids

The four small parathyroid glands are located in the neck at the base of the thyroid gland. They regulate the amount of calcium secreted into the bloodstream, reserved in the bones or excreted from the body. If calcium levels in the blood fall, the glands release parathormone which does the following:

• Signals the kidneys to put calcium back into the bloodstream rather than excreting it through the urine.

• Activates Vitamin D allowing the intestines to absorb more from the foods we eat.

• Stimulates the breakdown of bone to release stored calcium into the bloodstream.

Calcium-Phosphorus Imbalance

The blood desires a ratio of 2.5 parts calcium to 1 part phosphorus. Parathormone is stimulated by phosphorus. When there is excess phosphorus in the blood stream, parathormone signals the body to pull calcium out of the bones and tissues to achieve that ratio. The proper ratio for bones is about 2.2 parts calcium to 1 part phosphorus.

Too Much Phosphorus

Americans have doubled their daily intake of phosphorus in the last 40 or 50 years. Phosphorus is found in carbonated beverages and is added to processed foods like meats, cheese, and bread.

Calcium deficiency in the bloodstream causes the parathyroid glands to secrete parathormone that tells the calcium in the bones to be released into the blood.

Phosphorus Interference: Antacids

Antacids impair gastrointestinal phosphorus absorption. Long term or regular use of antacids (containing magnesium hydroxide and/or aluminum hydroxide) can cause phosphorus to be depleted in the blood. This decreases the absorption of calcium which can result in the loss of skeletal calcium and phosphorus.

Antacid Scam

Many antacids claim in their marketing literature to be *"a good source of calcium."* What good is this calcium if you cannot absorb it? Tums, Rolaids, and other antacid products contain calcium carbonate, which actually is **chalk**, and of all available forms of calcium, is the least well absorbed. Studies show that most calcium supplements simply do no good for individuals suffering from bone loss.

Many individuals use antacids to diminish stomach acid. But stomach acid is required for the breakdown and absorption of the calcium.

Next to aspirin, more people use more antacids than any other over-the-counter drug. The truth is they are ruining your bones.

Aluminum

We have known for some time that antacids containing aluminum cause calcium loss as a consequence of phosphorus depletion and may contribute to the development of skeletal demineralization. (Spencer, Goyer) But remember, aluminum is found in many other things which we encounter daily: antiperspirants, soft drink and beer cans, foil wrap, many medications and is a common additive in our food and water. We do indeed absorb aluminum from these sources. (Kohara)

Inefficient Calcium Absorption

Inability to absorb sufficient calcium through the intestines can cause a calcium deficiency. Adequate stomach acid is required for calcium absorption. As we grow older, we produce less stomach acid making it more difficult for us to absorb calcium.

Certain substances in some foods make it more difficult to absorb the calcium in our diet. These include spinach, rhubarb and foods with a high fiber content.

Calcium is absorbed through the intestinal tract, and fiber shortens the time that our food travels through the intestinal tract. The less time the food is there, the less time we have to absorb calcium, other minerals, and other nutrients as well. While a high fiber diet has many advantages, with too much fiber this is one disadvantage. However, many people who may **think** they eat a "high" fiber diet may actually **not** be eating enough fiber to have a significant impact on calcium absorption. The high amount of processed foods in our diets has greatly decreased our fiber intake. If this is a concern for you, avoid eating high fiber foods at the same time as calcium-containing foods or supplements.

Vitamin D Deficiency

Among elderly individuals who experience hip fractures, 10 to 20% have impaired bone mineralization due to vitamin D deficiency. 800 IU of vitamin D is recommended daily. Vitamin D is needed to assimilate calcium, phosphorus, and magnesium. Vitamin D deficiency in children causes bone abnormalities known as rickets. In adults, vitamin D deficiency causes osteomalacia, which means "soft bones." Elderly patients with hip fractures at Massachusetts General Hospital in Boston checked for vitamin D levels revealed that all 142 individuals had low levels. In addition, 75% had osteomalacia, (Appleton)

Elevated Glucose

Diabetics tend to have a reduced bone density and higher incidence of osteoporosis than age-matched controls. Elevated sugar in the blood tends to depress calcium absorption in the intestinal tract. Over time this is sure to take its toll.

As we grow older, insulin, the hormone which carries glucose into the cells to be burned, becomes less effective. This is termed insulin resistance. A primary cause of insulin resistance is chromium deficiency. Insulin cannot do its job without chromium. Scientists at the United States Department of Agriculture (USDA), including Dr. Gary Evans, Ph.D., found that diets high in simple sugars trigger loss of chromium through the urine, which can further the problem of insulin resistance.

When cells are resistant to insulin and insulin levels are high, another problem arises. DHEA production decreases. This is highly significant in post-menopausal women because their production of estrogen via the reproductive tract has practically stopped and the body relies upon healthy DHEA levels. DHEA converts into estrogens. Diminished estrogen levels also contribute to calcium loss.

Dr. Evans reports that a daily supplement of 200 mcg. Chromium significantly reduced calcium loss in the urine, and increased levels of DHEA and estrogens in postmenopausal women. (Evans)

Alcohol and Caffeine

Alcohol and caffeine containing beverages are natural diuretics which cause us to eliminate increased amounts of urine and increased amounts of calcium, magnesium and sodium.

A 5 oz. cup of brewed coffee or tea may contain between 45 and 80 mg. of caffeine. A 12 oz. serving of a carbonated soft drink (reg or diet) contains between 36 and 55 mg. caffeine. A serving of chocolate contains between 4 and 20 mg. caffeine, and who can eat one serving of chocolate?

With three cups of caffeinated coffee, 45 mg. of calcium is excreted into the urine.

In a group of postmenopausal women with reduced bone densities, it was found that 31 percent of the women drank 4 or more cups of coffee a day. In a group of women with normal bone density, only 3 percent drank that amount of coffee.

Many prescription and non-prescription drugs contain high levels of caffeine. Following are just a few:

	Mg Caffeine per tablet
Cafergot (for migraines)	100
Darvon (pain reliever)	32.4
Fiorinal (for headaches)	40
Appedrine (for weight control)	100
Codexin (for weight control)	200
Dex-A-Diet II (for weight control)	200
Diatac (for weight control)	200
No Doz (for alertness)	100
Vivarin (for alertness)	200
Exedrin (headaches/pain reliever)	65
Midol (PMS/pain reliever)	32.4
Aqua-Ban Plus (diuretic)	200
Permathene	200
Triaminicin (cold & allergies)	30
Coricidin-D (cold remedy)	30

Tobacco

Women who smoke reach menopause an average of five years sooner than non-smokers. Cigarette smoking has been shown to stop estrogen activity. Cigarette smoke contains a number of toxic substances including hydrozine and cadmium. So not surprisingly, smoking is also associated with increased cadmium exposure. Cadmium causes calcium to be pulled from the bone and excreted.

Cadmium is a mineral used in the manufacturing of batteries, plastics, paints, and fertilizers. Excessive exposure to cadmium has an adverse effect on blood pressure, the kidneys and bones. In addition to cigarette smoke, significant sources include motor oil, tires and galvanized parts of motor vehicles.

Smoking is also associated with a vitamin B-6

deficiency which is depleted by exposure to hydrozine compounds in cigarette smoke. (Roepke)

Lack of Exercise

Exercise plays a critical role in our overall health and well being. Exercise increases our bone strength. Lack of use, as well as weightlessness causes our bones to become weaker as they experience diminished density.

An Australian study on the prevention of postmenopausal osteoporosis using 120 postmenopausal women with low forearm bone density in a double-blind, placebo-controlled study compared several treatment combinations by measuring changes in the distal and medium forearm. They found significant bone loss in the group with normal bone density (control group) and the exercise group (change, respectively). Bone loss was significantly lower in the exercise-calcium group, and bone density increased at this site in the exercise-estrogen group.

The researchers concluded that in postmenopausal women with low bone density, bone loss can be slowed or prevented by exercise plus calcium supplementation or estrogen-progesterone replacement. Although the exercise-estrogen regimen was more effective than exercise and calcium supplementation in increasing bone mass, it also caused more side effects. (Prince, 1991)

Protein ... Too Much/Too Little

Excess protein is one of the major problems of the typical American diet. Excessive dietary protein promotes bone loss as calcium excretion increases.

21

Calcium is mobilized out of the bones to buffer the increased acidity caused by the high protein.

In addition, the amino acid methionine is converted to homocysteine which appears also to encourage bone loss. The major dietary sources of methionine are animal proteins such as meat, chicken, fish, eggs, and dairy products. While this amino acid is an essential nutrient, excess amounts can cause problems with the health of your bones.

Vegetarian diets which provide less protein (and methionine) than the typical American diet are associated with healthier bones in postmenopausal women. (Marsh) However, strict vegetarian diets may not provide an adequate source of vitamin D, which is of great importance to bone health.

Vitamin B-6

Vitamin B-6 supplementation has shown to help prevent osteoporosis for a number of reasons. Vitamin B-6 is a cofactor necessary for strong structural protein connective tissue in bones. Vitamin B-6 also may influence the production or activity of progesterone. (Roepke) Vitamin B-6 also reduces harmful homocysteine levels which increase in women around the time of menopause. Homocysteine encourages bone loss.

Menopausal women are also at high risk for a vitamin B-6 deficiency. Risk for bone loss is much higher in individuals with a vitamin B-6 deficiency. (Reynolds) Animal studies show that a Vitamin B-6 deficiency caused impaired bone growth and repair, and were at a higher risk for development of osteoporosis. (Benke, Dodds)

Vitamin B-6 deficiencies are more prevalent today than one would expect and are even more common among older individuals. Thanks to today's modern society we have chemicals (such as hydrazines found in some food dyes, herbacides, plant growth regulators, food preservatives, etc.) which interfere with B-6 action in the body. Even if we manage to obtain the governments low RDA of just 2 mg, (and many people do not), this may not be enough, thanks to these chemicals floating around in our food and water.

Because of the safety of low dose supplementation of B-6, 5-25 mg daily is recommended. Because B-6 works with magnesium, you may wish to consider also supplementing magnesium to ward off any potential, but unlikely, side effects such as insomnia and irritability. Some individuals (with asthma, carpal tunnel syndrome or PMS) may wish to take 50 to 100 mg B-6 daily. (Gaby)

Hormone Imbalance

Hormones are like little messengers reporting to the rest of the body. Each hormone essentially has a different message. When there are proper levels of all hormones circulating in the body, everything is in order.

Osteoporosis is associated to an altered secretory response of parathyroid glands maybe due to reduced sensitivity of the parathyroid cells to extracellular calcium. (Rubinacci)

Corticosteriod Hormones

Corticosteriods, such as Prednisone, prescribed for inflammatory conditions such as arthritis, lupus, asthma, emphysema, etc., inhibits calcium gastrointestinal absorption. Because these conditions are usually chronic, long term treatment is common and the result is increased prevalence in bone loss and increased incidence of fractures compared to age-matched controls.

Estrogen Dominance

Estrogen dominance is one of the newer theories in osteoporosis ideology and is not (yet) fully accepted by all medical professionals. I am not telling you this because it has less validity than the other causes, I am warning you that if you bring up the subject with your health care practitioner, he or she may not have a clue to what you are talking about.

Because of the abundance of environmental pseudo-estrogens in western civilized societies we are bombarded with estrogens creating an imbalance with our other hormones, primarily progesterone.

Estrogen replacement therapy (unopposed estrogen without progesterone), hysterectomy, birth control pills, exposure to xenoestrogens and dietary abundance all contribute to estrogen dominance. Excess calories with an abundance of animal fats, sugars, refined starches, and processed foods lead to estrogen levels in women twice as high as women in third-world countries. This sets the stage for an exaggerated estrogen decline at menopause. (Lee)

If you eat meat, I strongly recommend that you consume hormone-free meat as the testosterone given to these animals to promote growth breaks down into estrogen-like chemicals which can create imbalances in our hormone levels.

In addition to pre and post menopausal bone loss, other problems associated with estrogen dominance include: allergies, diminished sex drive, depression, fatigue, fibrocystic breasts, increased blood clotting, infertility, miscarriage, PMS, uterine cancer, uterine fibroids, fat gain (especially around the belly, hips, and thighs), autoimmune disorders such as lupus, and water retention.

Current Therapies

Menopause and the decreased production of estrogen and progesterone, the two main "female" hormones, has been associated with the increased risk for the development of osteoporosis. However, in spite of the evidence that estrogen and progesterone therapy may offer some benefit, I am not convinced that we understand the entire picture in regards to this situation. Postmenopausal osteoporosis primarily occurs in Western civilized women. The percentage of women and individuals experiencing problems with bone loss has greatly increased over the last several centuries.

In Africa, Bantu women demonstrate very little osteoporosis, even after menopause, which occurs at the same age as American women. However, Bantu women have much higher estrogen levels compared to American women following menopause. Why? Some researchers believe it is diet related. Bantu women consume a minimum of milk, sugar, caffeine, alcohol, or drugs. They consume no calcium supplements and no estrogen therapy.

Not all American women experience accelerated bone loss after menopause and there are risks associated with estrogen therapy. Therefore, hormone replacement therapy is not the answer for all women reaching menopausal age.

Osteoporosis is not caused by menopause, and it

is not caused by an estrogen deficiency. (If it were, all men would have osteoporosis, right?!) The pharmaceutical industry seems to have come up with this idea. Osteoporosis actually begins long before (five to 20 years before) estrogen levels fall during the menopausal years. Taking estrogen can slow bone loss for those few years, but this effect wears off a few years after menopause. (Lee)

Estrogen & Progesterone Replacement Therapy

While estrogen has shown to temporarily slow down the reabsorption of bone in postmenopausal women, and even reduce fractures by as much as 50%, it **does not** promote new bone growth. If estrogen supplementation stops, bone loss resumes, possibly at an accelerated rate. In order for estrogen therapy to prevent osteoporosis, it must begin before significant bone loss has occurred and must continue indefinitely. (Gaby)

Progesterone Benefits

Progesterone in combination with estrogen is believed by many to be superior to supplementing estrogen alone. Some studies have indicated that natural progesterone such as from wild yam are just as beneficial as synthetics, but with fewer side effects.(Lee)

Progesterone given alone to post-menopausal women has also shown promise to assist in the prevention of bone loss. Thirty-five early postmenopausal women who had not received any form of treatment to prevent bone loss were randomly assigned to a 2-year regimen of 500 micrograms/day of a progesterone (Promegestone) or a placebo for 21 days out of a 28-day treatment cycle.

Loss of bone mineral density in the placebo group after 2 years of treatment was average of 4.5%. In the progesterone group, the rate of bone change was significantly lower and urinary calcium excretion was lower. (Tremollieres)

Side Effects and Risks

Hormone replacement therapy using estrogen or a combination of estrogen and progesterone are not ideal because of the many health risks which increase with the use of these synthetic hormone analogs, including the increase for certain kinds of cancer.

In addition, replacement therapy with estrogen and progesterone prevents bone loss for only a short period of time. After a few years, bone loss continues at the same rate that it was previous to the replacement therapy.

The possible side effects and definite increased health risks associated with synthetic hormone replacement therapy include:

Uterine and breast cancer
Gall bladder disease
Blood clots
Fluid retention
Weight gain
Breast tenderness
Depression
Skin breakouts
Alopecia (hair loss)
Masculizing - body hair, deep voice
Depression
Nausea and dizziness

Insomnia or sleepiness
Spotting, amenorrhea
Rise in blood pressure
Migraine headaches
Nervousness
Changes in sex drive

DHEA

DHEA, which stands for dehydroepiandros-terone, the "mother" hormone produced in our adrenal glands, has been shown to improve osteoporosis through a number of mechanisms. (Mayer) DHEA has a direct effect on both resorption and formation of bone. DHEA can also increase the levels of other major hormones - estrogen, progesterone, and testosterone, important for bone mineral density. Men who have low levels of testosterone have a higher incidence of osteoporosis.

In a study of postmenopausal women, administering DHEA increased serum levels of both testosterone and estrogens. (Regelson)

Administration of DHEA to ovariectomized rats significantly increased bone mineral density. These findings strongly suggest that serum adrenal androgen may be converted to estrogen, and be important steroids to maintain bone mineral density, especially after menopause in the sixth to seventh decades. (Nawata)

How DHEA Prevents Bone Loss

1. DHEA improves calcium absorption, possibly due to effects on vitamin D metabolism.

2. A breakdown product of DHEA binds to estrogen receptors. Therefore DHEA, like estrogen, inhibits bone resorption.

3. Androgens (which include DHEA and testos-terone) stimulate bone formation and calcium absorption. DHEA might, therefore, augment the bone-building effect of progesterone. DHEA appears to be the only hormone capable of inhibiting bone resorption AND stimulating bone formation.

4. DHEA plays an important role in maintaining bone mass in postmenopausal women. In pre-menopausal women with Addison's disease (adrenal insufficiency), enough DHEA is apparently made by the ovaries to compensate for the weak adrenal glands. This most likely explains why these women do not develop osteoporosis. After menopause, how-ever, when ovarian production of DHEA and other hormones slows down, if the adrenal glands are not capable of taking over, a marked deficiency of DHEA results. It is quite possible that giving DHEA to post-menopausal women with adrenal insufficiency would prevent the accelerated bone loss that these women experience.

DHEA and Calcium Metabolism

Experiments performed almost 20 years ago by Dr. Hollo, a Hungarian researcher, showed that plas-ma levels of DHEA-S were significantly lower in post-menopausal women with osteoporosis than in matched controls. He also found another abnormali-ty in these women; when given calcium by intra-venous injection, the calcium level in their blood-stream remained elevated for an unusually long peri-od of time. However, after a week receiving oral DHEA-S (100 mg/day) their calcium metabolism returned to normal, suggesting that the body is making use of it. (Hollo)

Several series of data suggest that alterations in adrenal androgen output might be a contributing factor to changes in bone mass. The possible relationship between bone density and serum levels of DHEA was examined in 105 women (aged 45-69 years; 76 postmenopausal, 29 premenopausal).

Serum DHEA level was significantly lower in the individuals with low bone density. The serum DHEA level decreased significantly with age among all individuals. After correcting for age, there was a significant positive relationship between DHEA and mineral density of the bones of the lower spine, neck, and arm. Since there was no significant difference between the two groups regarding estrogens, this study suggests that DHEA may have a non-oestrogenic effect on bone. (Szathmari)

Drug Therapies

When a significant amount of bone mass has been lost, therapeutic drug interventions are aimed at preventing further loss with use of antiresorptive agents (ie, estrogen, progestin, calcitonin, and bisphosphonates). Use of pharmacologic agents that stimulate bone formation is still in experimental stages.

Bisphosphonates are synthetic compounds similar to pyrophosphate in the body which is composed of phosphorus and carbon.

Bisphosphonates (such as etidronate) are currently used in the management of patients with osteoporosis. They are taken up preferentially by the skeleton and suppress bone resorption by binding to existing hydroxyapatite crystals.

Studies show that long term therapy with oral bisphosphonates does not affect the calcium response for individuals with very low calcium levels with osteoporosis. (Landman)

The dosage of Bisphosphonates needed to inhibit bone resorption impairs the mineralization of newly synthesized bone matrix so long term administration would not be feasible. Bisphosphonates are poorly absorbed so may cause gastrointestinal irritation. In 1992 the Drug Therapy review in the *New England Journal of Medicine*, Drs. Lawrence Riggs and L. Joseph Melton suggested the therapy may be more beneficial when a 2 week regimen of etidronate be alternated with 11 to 13 weeks of calcium supplementation. The researchers also pointed out that prevention was the best treatment for osteoporosis. (Riggs, 1992)

Adendronate Sodium is a new bisphosphonate drug prescribed to postmenopausal women diagnosed with osteoporosis. It is designed to reduce the activity of the cells which cause bone loss (osteoclasts). It is not recommended for women with difficulty swallowing, with certain disorders of the esophagus, stomach or digestion, for those with low calcium blood levels, or kidney problems. It is also not recommended for pregnant women. Side effects include chest pain, severe difficulty or pain upon swallowing, abdominal pain and other less frequent effects: gas, bloating, constipation, diarrhea, muscle/bone pain. headache, altered taste and rash. (Merck)

Calcitonin (a thyroid hormone which inhibits bone resorption) levels tend to decrease with advancing age. There is some evidence linking lower calcitonin levels with osteoporosis. Synthetic calcitonin (Calcimar) has been approved by the FDA for treatment of postmenopausal osteoporosis but it is very expensive (about $7.50 a day or $2,700 a year). It is injected daily either into the muscle or under the skin. Side effects include nausea, vomiting, transient facial flushing, and inflammation at the injection sight. Calcitonin has caused severe allergic reactions and at least one death. (Gaby) (Riggs. 1992)

Calcium
Just one part of the story

The greatest misconception about osteoporosis is probably the belief that it is due to a lack of dietary calcium. While calcium has great importance to healthy bones, one must not forget to examine the causes of the lost calcium and calcium displacement from bone (resorption).

Calcium is the most abundant mineral in the body. The main function of calcium is to act in cooperation with phosphorus to build and maintain bones and teeth. It is also essential for healthy blood, helps regulate the heartbeat, is needed for nerve and muscle stimulation and for blood clotting processes. Calcium absorption normally requires strong stomach acid secretions and usually only about 20 percent is absorbed.

Ninety-nine percent of the body's entire calcium content is found in the skeleton. Soft tissues and blood contain the remaining.

Calcium is the major structural mineral in bone. A severe lack of calcium threatens bone health by creating a negative calcium balance, where more calcium is withdrawn from bone to meet the body's other calcium requirements than is being replaced. Simply increasing calcium intake does not guarantee strong bones. No nutrient functions in isolation. Studies have shown conclusively that neither calcium supple-

ments nor high calcium diets can do much more than
slow bone loss down somewhat.

Foods High in Calcium

Milk and milk products, fish, eggs, cereal products, beans, many types of nuts and seeds, fruit
(especially oranges and papaya), and vegetables
(especially green leafy) are high in calcium.
Meat contains calcium, but like dairy products, is
not a good source to rely upon because its protein
and phosphorus content actually contribute to calcium loss.
"Calcium fortified" foods are abundant and can
be found in foods ranging from breakfast cereals to
soup to orange juice.

	Calcium (approx.)
Low fat yogurt (plain) -1 cup	420 mg.
Low fat yogurt (fruit flavored) -1 cup	350 mg.
Sardines (canned) - 3 oz.	372 mg.
Skim milk -1 cup	300 mg.
Sesame seeds -1 tablespoon	300 mg.
Calcium fortified orange juice - 8 oz.	300 mg.
Calcium fortified cereal -1 cup	300 mg.
Cheese (cheddar, colby, etc.) -1 oz.	220 mg.
Figs -10 dried	270 mg.
Mackerel - 3 oz, canned	200 mg.
Farina, enriched (instant, cooked) -1 cup	190 mg.
Greens (turnip, collard, mustard) -1/2 cup	120-170 mg.
Salmon (canned) -3 oz.	165 mg.
Almonds -1/2 cup	160 mg.

Broccoli (cooked)-1 cup	140 mg.
Blackstrap molasses -1 tablespoon	140 mg.
Tofu (processed with calcium) - 4 oz.	140 mg.
Soybeans (cooked) -1 cup	130 mg.
Rhubarb -1 cup	120 mg.
Shrimp -1 cup	80 mg.
Orange -1 medium	60 mg.
Corn tortilla -1 medium	60 mg.
Beans (cooked, kidney, navy, etc.) -1/2 cup	45 mg.
Egg - 1 large	27 mg.

Calcium Facts:

* The human body contains about 1,100 grams of calcium. This makes up about 1.5 % of our total body weight.

* Calcium, as the primary structural mineral in bone, is essential for skeletal health. In addition, the one percent of our body's supply not found in bone is likewise critical to the heart, muscles, nerve function, and metabolic processes.

* 80 percent of all American women are calcium deficient.

* Men and women over age 30 require up to 67 percent more calcium than do 16 year olds.

* According to "The Calcium Bible" by Patricia Hausman, M.S., calcium is not only essential as a bone-building nutrient, but also shows promise as one which helps control blood pressure. The Calcium Information Center reports that blood pressure can be reduced by increasing calcium intake.

* Calcium is important to assist in vitamin

absorption as well as help with nerve, hormone and enzyme functioning.

* Some research findings reveal the most effective time to supplement calcium is nighttime. However, at this time, if you have an empty stomach, you may wish to also supplement betaine hydrochloride to assist in absorption.

* Other studies report that calcium mineral supplements should be taken with food because the stomach will naturally produce hydrochloric acid at that time. The best advice may be to take your calcium supplement 2 to 3 times per day as it is believed that the body can only absorb about 500 mg calcium at a time.

* The form of the calcium taken and which co-nutrients it is taken with are important in achieving the most beneficial results from a calcium supplement. Vitamin D (particularly D-3) is needed for optimal calcium absorption.

One of the basic principles of nutrition is that no nutrient ever works alone. Calcium is by no means an exception to this rule.

Assimilation

Calcium absorption and assimilation by the body is not always easy. Calcium we take in through foods or various supplements won't do us much good if it cannot be easily digested or assimilated. And once it enters the blood stream, its value will be limited by the availability of important calcium co-factors. We cannot hope to maintain or restore strong, healthy bones without them.

Proper stomach acidity is required for calcium to

dissolve. If you are not sure you have adequate stomach acidity, try taking your calcium supplement with 1 tablespoon vinegar mixed with 1 tablespoon honey or with a hydrochloric acid supplement. Sometimes it may be better to chew the tablets to help break them down.

Does your calcium tablet dissolve?

Not in a glass of water, but in a glass of vinegar at room temperature. Stir it around a few times and after 30 minutes the tablet should dissolve into fine particles. If not, the tablets would probably have a hard time dissolving in your stomach and are pretty much useless.

In a similar test of 21 commercial calcium products, 11 brands failed. (Shangraw) When shopping for a good calcium/mineral supplement, don't let marketing hype and price convince you. The least expensive brand may not be the best buy if you do not assimilate any of the calcium, and the most expensive brand may just be an attempt to entice you to pay for a lot of misleading advertising claims.

Calcium Co-factors

In order to absorb and assimilate calcium as well as other important minerals for good bone health (phosphorus and magnesium), vitamins A, D, and C are necessary.

A diet too high or too low in cholesterol makes it difficult for the body to assimilate the fat soluble vitamins A and D.

Vitamin D mineralizes the skeleton by elevating calcium and phosphorus in the blood. It does this by working with the parathyroid hormone to stimulate absorption in the intestinal tract and to increase renal reabsorption of calcium in the distal tubules. (Yamamoto)

As we grow older, our ability to produce vitamin D diminishes. (Tanaka) There is an abundant amount of evidence that suggests that vitamin D -3 supplementation (4,000 IU daily) would aid postmenopausal women with osteoporosis, however, the clinical trials do not support this. (Christianson, Ott-1989)

Larger amounts (7,500 IU daily) have shown better results but are associated with the increased risk of hypercalcemia and hypercalciuria. (Aloia)

We all can benefit from an absorbable calcium/ mineral formulation, especially those most vulnerable to bone loss; women during and past menopause, anyone with questionable diets or sedentary lifestyles, and senior citizens (men included).

Milk and the Calcium Controversy

If you think milk and dairy products are good for your bones you have been one of the millions who believe what the media and the daily industry would like us to.

Milk may create calcium deficiency and weaken bones. Contrary to popular belief and what the dairy industry would like us to believe, the calcium in milk is not highly usable by the body, says a bulletin titled "*Milk, No Longer Recommended or Required*" from the Physicians Committee for Responsible Medicine (PCRN).

According to Dr. Neil Barnard, MD, President of PCRN, only 30 percent of the calcium in dairy products is absorbed. But, even more important, he warns, that athletes, especially body builders, have a very serious reason to avoid dairy products. "The animal protein in cow's milk causes calcium wastage and calcium loss from the bone. In 1981 the *Journal of Nutrition* had more than one report demonstrating the negative effect the sulphur-containing proteins in dairy products had on calcium and bone."

"Interestingly, plant protein does not seem to cause the same problems. If you look at the strongest known animals, the bull, oxen, horse, gorilla, and elephant, all with beautiful musculature and incredibly strong bones, they are all complete vegetarians. They have no need for tissue or dairy protein in their diets and yet support dense, strong muscles and bones," said Barnard.

According to Gary Null, nutritionist and author of *The Vegetarian Handbook*, the phosphorus contained in milk binds to the calcium making the calcium unusable, and most of it is excreted. He also points out that the high amount of protein (unneeded nonessential amino acids in casein) in milk results in excess urea, which has to be processed by the kidneys. The high concentration of the calcium mixed with the uric acid in the kidneys can create kidney stones. In addition, when the uric acid is excreted, it takes along with it, calcium and other minerals. This point was also made by nutritionist Suzanne Havala, MS, RD, at the PCRM Press Conference.

If the body becomes depleted in calcium, eventually the body will take it from the bones, rendering them weak and brittle. This disease, osteoporosis, has become very prevalent in the United States, and according to a number of authorities, the reason may lie in excess consumption of animal protein.

In 1987, the *Journal of Clinical Investigation* reported that dairy products have little effect on women with osteoporosis. According to *Science* (1986) there is a large body of evidence indicating no positive relationship between calcium intake and bone density.

Dr. John McDougall, MD, author of *The McDougall Plan*, says, "Unfortunately, the people in this country have the wrong message as to what the cause of this disease (osteoporosis) is. They believe (for a very good reason: multi-millions of dollars are spent convincing them) that osteoporosis is due to cow's milk deficiency."

According to Dr. William Ellis, MD, past president of the American Academy of Applied Osteopathy, blood tests show that people who drink three or four glasses of milk a day invariably had the lowest levels of blood calcium.

In addition, calcium is highly basic in pH which lowers the acidity of the hydrochloric acid in the stomach. (Milk is a common antidote for acid poison.) The cells which produce hydrochloric acid have to work harder to produce more to digest our food. Eventually these cells cannot keep up and slow down. Inadequate hydrochloric acid levels cannot completely digest proteins which can cause allergic reactions.

Dr. Frank Oski, author of the book *"Don't Drink Your Milk,"* points out an interesting point:

"Per quart, cow's milk contains about 1,200 mg calcium, while human breast milk contains about 300 mg calcium per quart, yet babies absorb more calcium from breast milk."

When I spoke with the famous "baby doctor," Dr. Benjamin Spock, M.D., about the calcium in cow's milk he pointed out that in most other countries in the world, adults do not drink milk at all, yet seem to have no problems with osteoporosis. He also stated that a number of studies show that supplementation with dairy products has no beneficial effect on calcium levels and osteoporosis.

In case you are wondering where you get your calcium if it's not from diary products...

A report in the *American Journal of Clinical Nutrition* (1990) reported that calcium from green leafy kale was more absorbable than calcium from milk. It turns out that vegetables are a very good source of usable calcium for the body. Broccoli, cauliflower, watercress, parsley, other leafy vegetables, and sea vegetables, are rich in absorbable calcium.

Sardines, anchovies, caviar, herring, salmon (especially Pacific), are very high in usable calcium. Scallops and shrimp also contain calcium.

Sesame seeds, almonds, hazelnuts, peanuts, pistachios, soy beans (and tofu), black beans, kidney beans, garbanzo beans, pinto beans, blackstrap molasses and many fruits (blackberries, currents, figs, goose berries, grapefruit, oranges, guava, papaya, rhubarb, etc.) are also excellent sources of calcium.

Vitamins A, D, and C are needed to absorb and assimilate calcium. Vitamins A and D are lost in the processing of milk and other dairy products, so they are added through fortification. However, dairy products contain no vitamin C.

Vitamin C is very important for calcium assimilation. That's why they started adding calcium to orange juice. Imagine! **We can now get more calcium benefits from drinking fortified orange juice than we can drinking milk!**

Lactose is also important for calcium absorption. If you are lactose intolerant and are consuming dairy products with the lactose removed, you are further decreasing the amount of calcium you can utilize.

Calcium More Bioavailable From Water than Milk

One study shows using 15 lactose intolerant male individuals, compared calcium bioavailability from a calcium-rich water verses milk. The study reported that the bioavailability of calcium from the water was generally as good as or better than that from milk. In eight of 15 subjects, there was a higher level of calcium absorption from mineral water than from milk; bioavailability was equal in five of 15 subjects. The potential implications of this observation for the prevention and management of age-related bone loss are important for preventive medicine and indicate a new, important source of dietary calcium for lactose intolerant individuals. (Halpern)

Calcium Supplements

The majority of calcium supplements sold today are garbage. Many of them are composed of calcium carbonate, which is chalk. This is the cheapest form of calcium. It is hard-to-digest and is often poorly absorbed, especially by the older half of the population. Most forms of calcium are believed to be better absorbed when taken on a full stomach because hydrochloric acid is secreted after we eat which can help absorption.

% of Calcium in Calcium Compounds

	% of Ca	Grams of compound to provide 1 gram of Ca
Calcium carbonate	40	2.5
Calcium oxide	50	2
Calcium phosphate	30	3.3
Bone powder	32	3
Microcrystalline Hydroxyapatite	23	4.3
Calcium citrate	21	4.8
Calcium lactate	13	7.7
Calcium gluconate	10	10
Calcium aspartate	9	10.1

Calcium Carbonate Less Effective Than Calcium Citrate

It is often suggested that the women who were most likely to benefit from calcium supplementation were those with low calcium intakes. In a double-blind, placebo-controlled, randomized trial to determine the effect of calcium on bone loss from the spine, femoral neck, and radius in 301 healthy post-menopausal women. Half of the women had a low calcium intake (below 400 mg per day), and the other half had a moderate intake (400 to 650 mg per day).

The women received either a placebo, 500 mg calcium carbonate or 500 mg calcium citrate malate per day for two years.

In women who had undergone menopause five or fewer years earlier, bone loss from the spine was rapid and was <u>not affected by supplementation with calci-</u>

um. In the postmenopausal women (six years or more) and those who were given the placebo, bone loss was less rapid in the group with the higher dietary calcium intake. In those with the lower calcium intake, calcium citrate malate prevented bone loss during the two years of the study; its effect was significantly different from that of placebo. Calcium carbonate maintained bone density at the femoral neck.

Women who were postmenopausal for six years or more with the higher calcium intake, all three treatment groups maintained bone density at the hip and radius and lost bone from the spine.

The study showed that healthy older postmenopausal women with a daily calcium intake of less than 400 mg can significantly reduce bone loss by increasing their calcium intake to 800 mg per day. At the dose tested, supplementation with calcium citrate malate was more effective than supplementation with calcium carbonate. (Dawson-Hughes)

Side Effects from Calcium Supplements

The most common side effects from calcium supplements is constipation and gas. Bone meal may contain toxic metals like lead. Many people are allergic or intolerant to calcium lactate.

I would have to say that the most serious side effect of supplementing most calcium supplements is bone loss. **That's right. Most of them just don't work!** Especially if taken alone, without other minerals needed for healthy bones.

I contacted the Calcium Information Center and unfortunately "mainstream" organizations are still misinforming the public by recommending calcium carbonate. They state that calcium carbonate contains the highest amount of elemental calcium, and claim that it is the most cost effective. But if it is not doing a bit of good, how can it be considered cost effective?

Calcium Deficiency

Calcium deficiency can lead to nervousness, fatigue, muscle cramping, menstrual problems, periodontal disease, high blood pressure, and yes, osteoporosis.

An adequate calcium intake is, without question, required for sound bone integrity. The skeleton actually serves as a storehouse for calcium, a "calcium bank," if you will.

Systemic calcium needs are so critical that the body will not hesitate to make withdrawals from our bank account when calcium levels in the blood fall too low. We use up and excrete a certain amount of calcium each day. If this is not replaced, the result is a "negative calcium balance" and steady loss of the mineral from our bones.

Bone IS NOT built by Calcium Alone!

Can osteoporosis be combatted by simply gobbling more calcium? Research suggests otherwise. In fact, nutritional scientists such as Dr. Jeffrey Bland, are coming to the conclusion that bone loss is not a calcium problem at all.

One study published in the *New England Journal of Medicine* looked at the effect of calcium supplementation on 43 postmenopausal women and found "no effect on trabecular bone." Trabecular bone is the soft bone in the skeletal areas where osteoporosis starts.

Scientists have also studied individuals such as the Bantu in Africa who eat relatively calcium-poor diets. Surprisingly, the incidence of osteoporosis among these groups is strikingly low.

Consuming mainly whole grains and unrefined foods, they do get plenty of magnesium and trace minerals. Magnesium is the key which opens the door for calcium to be absorbed by bone.

Calcium Alone Offers No Benefit

A two year study with middle-aged women who had severe osteoporosis combined 500 mg of calcium per day orally with 0.5 mg of synthetic calcitonin (a hormone which inhibits bone resorption) subcutaneously three times per week. This resulted in a significantly increased calcium absorption rate. Their serum calcium and urinary Ca/Cr ratio increased somewhat. However, there was no evidence that the combined treatment improved the bone density. The calcitriol, instead of increasing the effect of calcitonin by suppression of the parathyroid, might have counteracted its effect by increasing the bone resorption. (Eriksson)

Several other studies suggest that calcium supplementation alone may have little to no benefit for postmenopausal women. (Gambacciani, Hasling) Women receiving hormone replacement therapy in conjunction with calcium supplementation had the best results compared to either approach by itself. These women experienced the largest increase in spinal bone mass, or least evidence of bone resorption. (Hasling)

One 3-year study with hormone replacement

therapy demonstrated that women still experience bone loss, however it was felt by the researchers that the hormone replacement therapy slowed the amount of loss. (Stevenson)

Other Minerals Found in Healthy Bones

Phosphorus is the second most abundant mineral in the body. It functions with vitamin D and calcium and is found in every cell in the body. It is essential for energy production, muscle contraction, digestion and the pH balance of the blood.

Food sources of phosphorus include meat, fish, poultry, eggs, whole grains, and seeds.

An intake of too much phosphorus can cause bone loss. This is highly prevalent in individuals who consume a diet high in animal protein.

Magnesium is an essential mineral found inside all cells where it is involved in many metabolic processes. The functions of magnesium include enzyme reactions, energy release (ATP), neuromuscular contraction, calcium absorption, protein synthesis and body temperature regulation. It also helps utilization of vitamin C, vitamin E, and the B Complex. Because magnesium is very alkaline, it helps regulate the acid-alkaline balance of the body.

Some experts believe that a calcium deficiency is actually caused by a magnesium deficiency which requires magnesium supplementation.

Magnesium is the key which opens the door for calcium to be absorbed by bone. Magnesium allows us to use our body's calcium supply more efficiently. Without magnesium, calcium builds up in soft tissues where it doesn't belong and cannot be incorporated into bone properly. Magnesium favors the hormonal mechanism that puts calcium back into bones. Experimental volunteers on magnesium-depleted diets, who were given calcium supplements, became deficient in calcium, in one research study. When the subjects were given magnesium, their calcium levels rose within a few days. The message is: Calcium must have magnesium as its partner in order to work.

Food sources of magnesium include fresh green vegetables, soybeans, unprocessed whole grains, seafood, figs, corn, apples, and almonds

Manganese is vital to the development of bones, ligaments, nerves and also is important to proper digestion. It is also important in sex hormone and milk production and functions as a catalyst and enzyme activator. Recent studies show a manganese deficiency contributes to excess blood sugar.

Manganese is found in whole-grain cereals, egg yolks, nuts, seeds, and green vegetables. **NOTE:** A great deal of manganese is lost in the processing and milling of foods.

Zinc is essential for proper bone maintenance. Bone tissue contains about 200 mcg. per gram of zinc. Several studies report that the average American diet only provides only 46-63% of the RDA for zinc. (Am. J. Clin Nutr., 1982)

Copper is needed for bone development and for mineralization and for hemoglobin function. It is also critical for healthy joints. About 19% of the body's copper is found in bone tissue.

Flouride and **sodium** are among the many trace elements necessary for mineralization. These minerals act as "mortar" giving bone hardness, strength and rigidity.

Silica, a trace mineral, is necessary for bone elasticity. When a baby is born, the ratio of calcium to silica is very different from the ratio of an older person. This may be why babies' bones are so resilient. With the loss of silica as bones become older, they become more brittle.

This is in accord with one of the conclusions of the osteoporosis symposium, which demonstrated that changes in the elasticity of bone result in a greater propensity to fracture. Bone growth involves the process of adding calcium for hardness, plus increasing collagen, the tough connective tissue that binds everything together and gives bones flexibility. Silica is essential for both these processes.

An important study conducted at the School of Public Health at the University of California, Los Angeles, (UCLA), shows that silica-supplemented bones have a 100 percent increase in collagen over low-silica bones. "If you do not have enough calcium and silica, your body leaches the calcium from your bones for tissue needs."

Silica is important in the following ways:

* In the formation and repair of bone, cartilage, skin and connective tissues of all kinds. Silica is an integral part of collagen and the protein complexes. It is crucial to the formation of bones and cartilage matrices.

* Participates in several metabolic processes.

* Required for calcification of bones in newborns.

* As a corrective dietary supplement in skeletal abnormalities resulting from silica deficiency.

Boron seems to play a role in the serum concentration of an estrogen hormone. In animals fed a boron deficient diet, bone abnormalities and growth problems developed. (Nielsen)

Bone Loss Is Not Inevitable

Fortunately for us, the body is an amazing structure and bone loss can be prevented. What's more, it is reversible. Lost bone can be restored. But calcium, important as it is for bone health, cannot do the job alone!

Researchers have taken a hard look at whether bone loss can be combatted by simply consuming large amounts of calcium, and have come up with some interesting and thought-provoking findings. The Bantu have been the focus of one landmark and often quoted study. Eating a diet high in whole grains, Bantus consume fairly little calcium. "Only a small minority are accustomed to daily intakes of more than 500 mg.", according to Dr. Alexander Walker, author of a report entitled; "Osteoporosis and Calcium Deficiency" (*American Journal of Clinical Nutrition*, Vol. 16, March 1965). 500 milligrams is much less than what most Americans get on a daily basis, with our high consumption of dairy foods, and far below the 1,500-2,000 mg. often recommended for bone health. All indicators point to a strikingly low incidence of bone disease among the Bantu, especially compared to those of us living in affluent western countries.

Clinical studies have been undertaken to determine if supplementation with calcium alone can do much to prevent bone loss. The verdict is negative. One trial reported in the New England Journal of Medicine found calcium supplementation had no effect on the soft, spongy bone found in places such as the spine, hip, wrist, and jaw–the most vulnerable areas.

All of this is leading nutritional scientists to the conclusion that bone loss is not just a calcium problem. Dr.Walker points out that bone loss consists of "reduction in bone mass ... without change in composition." Other researchers define bone loss as a condition "in which bone tissue is fully calcified, but there is too little of it." This means that all of bone's structural elements are lost when bone wastes away, not just the calcium.

If calcium alone is not the bone loss solution, then what is? To answer this, we need to understand more about the composition of bone. Bone is composed of a substance with a unique and intricate crystalline structure, called **microcrystalline hydroxyapatite, or 'MCHC**,' for short. Bone contains 67% hydroxyapatite by weight. Collegenous fibers make up the remaining 33%.

MCHC has been made available as a nutritional supplement to consumers following documented studies proving its immense value for bone health. MCHC contains not only calcium, but a number of other minerals as well: phosphorus, magnesium, and many important trace elements including manganese and silica. While the typical American diet is calcium-rich, it is often a poor source of trace minerals. The trace mineral content of commonly consumed food products, due to refining and processing, has seriously declined over the last fifty years or so.

MCHC Provides Bone Most Usable Form of Calcium

Unlike other calcium supplements, such as calcium carbonate and calcium gluconate, MCHC contains calcium in the actual form which is incorporated into bone. Bone is first formed as cartilage which is then mineralized. As bone matures the cartilage cells degenerate and disappear. Mineral salts (calcium, phosphorus, sodium and other trace minerals) replace the cartilage cells embedding themselves into the collagen matrix in the form of hydroxyapatite crystals. The mineral content of bone is continually turned over throughout life. About 18% of bone calcium turns over yearly in adults. In infants it turns over 100%.

Mineral Analysis of Healthy Bone

There are over 45 different minerals found in healthy bone tissue. All of these are found in microcrystalline hydroxyapatite, in their proper proportions.

Calcium
Phosphorus
Sodium
Magnesium

Silver
Tungsten
Boron
Copper

< 1 MG/GRAM
Zinc
Chloride
Strontium
Potassium
Barium
Aluminum

< 1 MCG/GRAM
Europium
Dysporsium
Ytterbium
Tantalum
Mercury
Uranium
Hafnium
Thorium
Silica

< 35 MCG/GRAM
Erbium
Arsenic
Iron
Bromine
Zirconium

< 100 NG/GRAM
Cobalt
Nickel
Platinum
Cesium
Lanthanum
Samarium
Terbium
Lutetium
Gold
Antimony
Indium
Iridium

< 10 MCG/GRAM
Neodymium
Gallium
Chromium
Scandium
Rubidium
Vanadium
Selenium
Manganese

Microcrystalline Hydroxyapatite (MCHC)

Microcrystalline hydroxyapatite (MCHC) is an extract from whole bone. It is identified chemically as $Ca_{10}(PO_4)_6(OH)_2$. It contains calcium, phosphorus, magnesium, and other important trace elements, but also features a lattice-shaped intricate crystalline structure which is of great clinical interest to bone specialists today.

This special network surrounds proteins such as collagen which make up the vital connective tissue holding us together. The living part of bone allows it to grow and to be rebuilt. These essential organic parts of bone tissue – contained in MCHC – are also lost as bone deteriorates, and must be replaced.

When bone loss occurs, all of these structural elements waste away. Osteoporosis has been defined as a condition in which "bone tissue is fully calcified and otherwise normal, except that there is too little of it." In other words, osteoporosis depletes all the stuff in bone, not just calcium.

How can one logically conclude that by supplementing calcium alone, that bone can be restored?

The secret to MCHC is that it not only contains the necessary calcium, but it also contains **ALL OTHER MINERALS and naturally occurring COMPONENTS found in bone** and in the **PROPER RATIO** that they naturally exist in bone.

MCHC Contains:

MINERALS:

Calcium is the most abundant mineral found in bone. MCHC contains on average about 24 % calcium by weight. Researchers agree that **MCHC** is an excellent source of bioavailable calcium. (Windsor, Epstein, Pines, Stephan)

Phosphorus is the second most abundant mineral in bone making up about 11% of its weight. It functions with vitamin D and calcium.

Magnesium. Allows us to use calcium more efficiently. Without magnesium, calcium builds up in soft tissues where it doesn't belong and cannot be incorporated into bone properly. Magnesium favors the hormonal mechanism that puts calcium back into bones. Calcium must have magnesium in order to work.

Manganese is vital to the development of bones, ligaments, and nerves.

TRACE MINERALS:

Fluoride (fluoroapatite), **Sodium, Zinc, Copper, Manganese, Boron, Nickel, Rubidium, Platinum, Strontium, Barium, Chloride, Potassium, and**

Silica. Deficiencies of any of these trace minerals which act as cofactors with enzymes needed to form the matrix can impair bone formation and resorption. (Saltman and Strause)

ACTIVE ENZYMES:
Including alkaline phosphatase. Special processing of MCHC is required to maintain the integrity of these raw enzymes. When looking for an MCHC supplement, make sure you purchase from a reputable company.

COLLAGEN PROTEIN:
Which make up about 23% by weight of the MCHC. The amino acids which make up this protein include hydroxyproline, glycine and glutamic acid.

MCHC Processing

Responsible MCHC manufacturers use young chemical free, freeze dried, bovine bones from range-grazed cattle to source their material. It is processed in a manner without high heat (called ashing) to preserve the constituents in their original physiological proportions and to preserve the delicate crystalline lattice. Not all manufactures will follow these important steps. Be sure to investigate to avoid heavy metals and other undesirables such as mad cow disease. No Mad Cow Disease is found in Australia or New Zealand, the two countries where MCHC is predominantly manufactured.

Bone meal and MCHC are not the same. Most bone meal is ashed, which yields a higher calcium content, but the protein collagens are destroyed. Bone meal has not clinically demonstrated to produce any benefits to individuals with osteoporosis. It is less expensive than MCHC. Only freeze-dried, non-ashed bone, called hydroxyapatite has shown the ability to increase bone mass.

Caution: Lead Contamination

Whenever considering supplementation of calcium products, it is important to examine the lead content. Lead contamination is widespread. Exposure to lead and other heavy metals contributes to intracellular accumulation of calcium where it does not belong.

Bone meal has reputation for lead contamination and it can also happen with MCHC so be sure that the brands you select are from a reputable manufacturer and that the product has been analyzed for lead content. Look for lead concentrations less than 2 parts per million.

MCHC: Amazing Ability to Restore Bone

MCHC has been proven to reconstruct and restore bone when taken as a supplement. No other calcium-type bone supplement has demonstrated this ability.

MCHC's remarkable bone-restoring powers are well documented in medical literature. Studies have demonstrated its effectiveness in cases of severe bone loss caused by liver disease and rheumatoid arthritis.

A study on the effect of MCHC whole-bone extract on absorption in the elderly demonstrated that MCHC was more efficiently absorbed than calcium gluconate. (Windsor)

In individuals with rheumatoid arthritis receiving corticosteriods, MCHC demonstrated the ability to slow bone loss. (Nilson)

A recent Swiss study published in 1995 evaluated whether ossein-hydroxyapatite (OHC) is more effective than calcium carbonate in preventing further bone loss in postmenopausal osteoporosis. Forty osteoporotic patients were monitored for 20 months. The patients were randomly assigned to one of two groups and treated in a double-masked manner with 1,400 mg calcium per day, in the form of either ossein-hydroxyapatite or calcium carbonate.

The bone densities were evaluated every 4 months. After 20 months of treatment the loss of trabecular bone was less in the ossein-hydroxyapatite group compared to the calcium carbonate group. This study shows that OHC is more effective than calcium carbonate in slowing peripheral trabecular bone loss in patients with manifest osteoporosis. (Ruegsegger)

MCHC Matrix Encourages Absorption

At least one study has demonstrated the significance of the matrix structure of MCHC. In a trial with osteoporosis patients, the effects of MCHC powder was compared to MCHC powder with the organic matrix destroyed by ashing. They found that the powder with the matrix intact was more successful in promoting calcium absorption and discouraging bone breakdown, even though the two preparations contained the same amount. (Durance)

MCHC More Effective than Calcium Gluconate

In a study to determine the effectiveness of MCHC compared to calcium gluconate, patients with osteoporosis were given MCHC with a small amount of DHT (dihydrotachysterol) over periods ranging from 8 months to 2 years. Bone density, which would otherwise normally decrease, was maintained over the entire period with MCHC supplementation of 8 grams daily. When the MCHC was replaced with calcium gluconate, the positive balance was reduced. While no adverse effects were noted with either supplement, the MCHC was more effective. (Dent)

MCHC Encourages Healing

The use of MCHC whole bone extract is useful for individuals with bone fractures. MCHC given to 127 patients in a double blind trial to investigate the healing effects of MHCH demonstrated healing (clinical union) of fractures in patients over age 55 at a rate of 3.2 weeks faster than controls who received no MCHC.

Individuals under age 55 who received treatment with MCHC had a more rapid healing time by 7 days compared to untreated controls. (Mills)

MCHC Safe (and effective) for Pregnant Women

According to the Calcium Information Center, a conservative organization who provides information regarding calcium nutrition and specific health care concerns, 1,500 to 2,000 mg of calcium daily can lower the risk of pregnancy-induced hypertension by 70% and the risk of preclampsia by over 60%.

In the special situation of pregnancy, most medications used for osteoporosis are contraindicated. Long-term heparin administration to treat deep thrombosis in the legs or pelvis may lead to substantial decreases in bone mass and consequently increased risk of osteoporosis. In an open randomized study, 9 women on heparin-treatment received daily 6.46 grams of hydroxyapatite-compound, over a period of 6 months and were compared to 11 women without bone protective treatment. In the hydroxyapatite-group, they experienced no side effects and reduced back pain. Bone mass did not change significantly, while it dropped significantly in the controls. (Ringe)

In other studies, MCHC was used for one month in 20 pregnant women at 28 to 40 weeks' gestation who were experiencing pain syndrome in the leg bones, lower back region who had disturbed dental status, and also on a second group of 13 women, with established clinically and roentgenologically climacteric osteoporosis. They took one pill daily for a period of 6 months. A considerable clinical improvement of pain syndrome and dental status was found in the end of the treatment in both groups. The positive therapeutic effect, ease of administration, tolerance and lack of side effects, make it convenient for treatment of disturbances in calcium-phosphorus balance. (Khadzhiev)

MCHC Slows Bone Loss Due to Corticosteroid Therapy - Reduces Pain

Long term use of corticosteriod hormones causes bone loss by reducing bone formation and by increasing bone breakdown (reabsorption) due to calcium malabsorption. To decrease bone reabsorption, hormones like estrogen and other anabolic steriods are often prescribed but have numerous risks and side effects and are contraindicated in individuals with chronic liver disease. MCHC supplementation is preferred because it is without side effects, and is perfectly safe for individuals with liver problems.

A controlled clinical trial carried out in 40 patients

at risk of osteoporosis because of long-term treatment with prednisone (5 to 20 mg/day) determined the ability of MCHC to prevent the appearance or progression of osteoporosis. Patients were treated with 6 to 8 grams of MCHC for 12 months and compared with the untreated control group. The two groups were well matched with regards to age, sex and underlying disease. The majority (68%) of the patients had back pain prior to the trial, the severity of which was graded at 3-monthly intervals. In the MCHC-treated group, there was a dramatic and significant reduction in pain during the trial, almost to the point of its disappearance. Of 19 patients with initial back pain only two still reported any pain at all after 12 months on the MCHC treatment. In the control group, back pain severity increased during the trial in three patients and was unchanged in the fourth.

Neither MCHC-treated, nor control group patients, showed any significant change in standing or stem height during the 12 month trial period. Both mean cortical thickness and mean metacarpal index figures showed small, insignificant decreases during the 12 months of the MCHC treatment but much more marked decreases in the control group. (Pines)

. In another study with patients with chronic active hepatitis (auto-immune) who were treated with corticosteriod therapy, MCHC supplementation also demon-

	CONTROL GROUP	MCHC GROUP
LOSS OF STEM HEIGHT	1.16 - 0.71 CM	0.87 - 0.58 CM
LOSS OF RADIAL BONE MINERAL CONTENT	0.056 - .033	0.043 - 0.029
LOSS OF RADIAL BONE DENSITY	5.29 - 3.34	4.78 - 3.5
SYMPTOMS WORSENED	11	4

strated reduced symptoms of osteoporosis. Individuals experienced reduced back pain and fractures, and a significant reduction in bone reabsorption. (Stellon) Individuals supplemented 8 grams a day of MCHC powder or tablets (which may seem a little high, but remember there has been no evidence of toxicity or side effects with use of MCHC), and these individuals were pleased with the results in spite of the inconvenience.

MCHC Increased Bone Thickness in Women with Chronic Liver Disease

MCHC was more effective than calcium gluconate in treatment of cortical bone thinning in postmenopausal women with primary biliary cirrhosis, a chronic liver disease which predominantly occurs in women.

Women with primary biliary cirrhosis had difficulty absorbing calcium, phosphate and vitamin D, and frequently develop accelerated cortical bone thinning. We have assessed the value of parenteral vitamin D, oral hydroxyapatite (MCHC), and calcium gluconate in the treatment of cortical bone thinning in primary biliary cirrhosis. Sixty-four postmenopausal women with primary biliary cirrhosis were assigned randomly into three groups: one group receiving no mineral supplements (control), one group receiving MCHC, and one group receiving calcium gluconate. All patients received parenteral vitamin D-2 (100,000 IU monthly).

Over a 14-month follow-up period, none of the groups showed a significant change in serum calcium or inorganic phosphate levels. Pre- and post-treatment hand radiographs were used to assess changes in metacarpal cortical thickness using the technique of caliper radiogrammetry. Cortical bone loss occurred in the control group. The MCHC group showed a significant gain in cortical bone thickness, while no significant change occurred in the calcium gluconate group. This study indicated that vitamin D-2 does not halt metacarpal cortical bone thinning in primary biliary cirrhosis. The addition of calcium gluconate prevents bone thinning, and MCHC promotes positive cortical bone balance. (Epstein)

MCHC Benefits Rheumatoid Arthritis

Corticosteriod hormones commonly prescribed for individuals with rheumatoid arthritis increases the risk for the development of osteoporosis.

In a 14 month study, individuals in the MCHC group received 6 grams daily. The MCHC group lost less stem height (seated height measured from crown to seat) compared to controls, and lost less radial bone mineral content than controls.

While loss of radial bone density comparisons were not considered to be of statistical significance, one can still see that the control group seemed to lose more than the MCHC group.

The researchers concluded that the MCHC was a valuable therapy in the prevention of osteoporosis in individuals with rheumatoid arthritis and suggested that MCHC be used concurrently with corticosteriods rather than waiting until osteoporosis has developed. (Nilsen)

Note: Recent research has revealed a **glucosamine sulfate** to be of great benefit to individuals with rheumatoid arthritis. Glucosamine sulfate provides the special mucopolysaccharides needed for healthy joint structure and for the fluid between the joints to maintain movement. Study results have been very promising. In one study with over 1,200 individuals, over 95% of those taking glucosamine sulfate experienced positive effects. (*Pharmatherapeutica* 1982, 3 (3): 157-168) See also *Current Research and Medical Opinion* 7(2):110-114 1980.

MCHC Prevents Bone Loss in Surgically-Induced Postmenopausal Women

After three years of supplementation with MCHC, postmenopausal women who were considered at risk for osteoporosis (they were already experiencing increased bone resorption), responded positively. They experienced fewer biological indications of bone resorption (urinary excretion of calcium and other minerals) and no further bone loss. (Stephan)

Additional Uses for Hydroxyapatite

Hydroxyapatite is presently under clinical investigation as a new biomaterial. It has been demonstrated to have potentially wide surgical application for use in reconstruction, periodontal disease, bone defects, orbital implants (the eye socket), and cranial reconstruction.

Hydroxyapatite Aids in Healing

Use of hydroxyapatite has shown to increase formation of woven bone in the healing process in the preparation for or during surgical implants. After several months, researchers could detect the hydroxyapatite was in intimate contact with the bone and later was partially included within its matrix. The hydroxyapatite granules applied allowed the implant to firmly embed into the existing area. The bone augmentation technique described has been used successfully in over 600 cases and is considered safe. (Remagen)

Hydroxyapatite has been used as a biologic "bone cement" in the reconstruction of suboccipital craniectomy defects. Within 2 years, cranial bone integrity can be reestablished. The frequency of debilitating postoperative headache was reduced in these patients when compared to patients who had no reconstruction defect. Reconstruction of the bony defect after surgery with hydroxyapatite cement is not only useful to restore cranial contour, but also appears to reduce some of the functional problems attributed to this surgical approach. (Kveton)

Interview with Dr. John Maher, D.C.

Doctors' View of MCHC On His Patients

To find out more about osteoporosis and the benefit of MCHC on patients experiencing bone loss, I spoke with Dr. John Maher, D.C., of Mission Valley Chiropractic, San Diego, CA (619) 298-0540.

Dr. Maher is a member of the following organizations: American Chiropractic Association, Californian Chiropractic Association, San Diego County Chiropractic Association, Foundation for Chiropractic R and D, ACA Council of Diagnostic Imaging. He has received numerous awards including Diplomat status from the American Academy of Pain Management and Best Chiropractor in San Diego. He has used MCHC as a part of his practice for the past five or six years and has seen impressive results in his practice in his patients experiencing pain due to primary osteoporosis.

Q: What is it about menopause which seems to stimulate bone loss in women?

Dr. Maher: During menopause, ovarian production of estrogen and progesterone dramatically slows or ceases causing a significant drop in the levels of these two hormones. Estrogen and progesterone in women are bone building. Estrogen inhibits osteoclast activity, which are the cells which stimulate the breakdown of bone. Progesterone supports osteoblastic activity.

The greatest amount of bone loss in women occurs 2 to 5 years after menopause. In men, osteoporosis is as common as it is in women, after the eighth decade. Androgen levels drop in men at a later age than female hormones in women.

Of course, changes in hormone levels, are not the only reasons why many people experience bone loss. The adrenal hormones (such as cortisol) which are associated with stress, are catabolic for bone. Any type of adrenal stimulant - weight loss drugs, caffeine, etc., is going to have a negative effect on the bones.

Q: Why is it that all women around the world do not experience bone loss after menopause?

Dr. Maher: Osteoporosis is primarily a disease seen in modern civilized industrialized countries. According to Dr. John Lee, M.D., author of *"Natural Progesterone"* and *"What Your Doctor May Not Tell You about Menopause,"* bones from women of comparable age from centuries ago had bone densities much higher than women of today. In third world countries today, osteoporosis is more rarely seen as the women seem to have a much higher bone density. Another interesting factor is that the calcium intake of these women is comparatively very low. Some authorities, like Dr. Lee, argue that the problem of bone loss is due to an estrogen dominance over progesterone. This estrogen dominance is suspected to largely be due to chemicals and petro-chemical products so prevalent in our "modern" society. These chemicals are also now known to affect bird and amphibian reproductive systems.

Certainly, there are other factors as well. We used to believe that the Japanese did not have a significant amount of cancer because of the their traditional low fat diet, however, it may actually be due to their high intake of soy foods which contain phyto-estrogens. These block estrogen receptor sights which is highly advantageous in an estrogen dominant, chemical environment.

Lack of exercise in our modern living is also a consideration.

Our high fat diet may also contribute to an estrogen dominant state.

Our high protein diet with high acid ash causes the body to alkalize it with calcium. The greatest reserve of calcium in the body of course is the bone tissue. It is believed by some authorities that if our protein intake were more "normal" the RDA for calcium would be closer to 500 mg compared to the 1500 mg that it is now.

Please keep in mind that osteoporosis is not a calcium deficient disease.

Other problem factors seen in "modern" diet are numerous; for example, our high intake of phosphorus, which is found abundantly in red meat and also in soda drinks. High phosphorus diets create a greater loss of calcium. Coffee, chocolate, cigarettes, alcohol, etc, are all detrimental to bone health.

Q: What are your views on milk and dairy consumption in regards to bone health?

Dr. Maher: Osteoporosis is not caused from not drinking enough milk. I believe that if a person is going to drink milk, it should be non-fat or low-fat. Cultured products are preferred because they have less lactose and have greater absorbability. They promote proper flora in the gut. This helps breakdown the lactate in dairy products. Of course, many people cannot tolerate milk products at all.

Because of our highly acidic diet (caused by phosphorus, protein and sugar), higher doses of calcium (800 to 1,500 mg) are needed daily. It may be difficult to obtain this amount of calcium without the use of dairy products (or usable supplements such as MCHC). Of course, dairy products are also high in protein so it is like a double-edge sword.

Q: Many cultures who do not consume milk and dairy products seem to have no problem with osteoporosis, correct?

Dr. Maher: Yes. African women of the Bantu region have been studied as they seem to have a very low incidence of osteoporosis. For the most part, they are vegetarians and do not drink milk. They do consume meat at feasts. Because, for the most part, they have no way to refrigerate, meat eating is not a regular component of their traditional diet.

Asians also do not particularly eat a lot of meat (using it primarily as a flavoring agent). They do not drink milk. Their daily calcium intake is about 400 to 500 mg of calcium. Yet, they do not experience the bone loss that women here in the US and Europe do.

Q: Vegetarians seem to have a lower incidence of osteoporosis as well?

Dr. Maher: In addition to the high protein, high phosphorus, high fat content problems with meat, industrialized meats also contain high amounts of petro chemicals. All of the petro chemicals used on our crops, etc. that we see in our environment end up in the fat of the animals at the top of the food chain. Rain washes these chemicals into our water systems which ultimately ends up in the ocean. Now the dolphins and whales are having great health (and reproductive) problems from this situation. Humans, of course, are at the very top of the food chain.

I would strongly recommend reading " A Diet for A New America" by John Robbins, who talks about how these chemicals become more concentrated the higher you climb up the food chain.

According to Dr. Lee, these petro chemicals promote estrogen dominance and hence, osteoporosis.

Q: Please tell us about MCHC and what you have seem in your practice in individuals with osteoporosis?

Dr. Maher: MCHC is microcystalline hydroxyapatite compound which comes from cattle bones. It contains the bone minerals calcium, phosphate, magnesium, fluoride, zinc, copper manganese, silica, rubidium, platinum, plus active enzymes, collagen, amino acids and other constituents all in the normal proportions as found in healthy bone.

I should point out that the bones used to manufacture MCHC should be from organically raised cattle, not exposed to hormones, pesticides, etc. New Zealand has been a reputable source to my knowledge.

The concept of giving someone with osteoporosis just calcium, or a supplement with calcium and a few other minerals really doesn't make much sense. Osteoporosis is actually a deficiency of the whole microcystalline structure of bone - this structure is what breaks down. We have seen that by supplying this structure, we can rebuild lost bone in secondary osteoporosis - that occurs as the result of taking drugs such as prednisone, biliary disease, etc.

We do know that the calcium in MCHC is absorbed better than any other calcium supplement.

Q: Why do you suspect that MCHC is superior than other "regular calcium supplements" or other "bone supplements"?

Dr. Maher: MCHC seems to have a superior affect on bone for a number of reasons. MCHC contains all of the components that make up healthy bone in the proper proportion. It contains live enzymes, collagen, trace minerals, and of course, the matrix microcrystalline structure.

A recent study in *Dynamic Chiropractic* discussed that supplementing trace minerals zinc, manganese and copper, builds better bones than supplementing calcium alone.

MCHC also contains fluoride in the form of hydroxy fluoride apatite compared to sodium fluoride (added to our drinking water). Sodium fluoride has negative effects on bone by making them more brittle, actually increasing hip fractures.

The proportion of these components of MCHC is of great significance. The studies conducted with MCHC used MCHC alone, not in combination with other nutrients. We are seeing a lot of new products containing MCHC in combinations recently, we really only know that MCHC is beneficial when taken **alone**. We don't really know if adding these things is benefiting the user or not. I would think that you would want to maintain the proportions. Also the product should contain authentic MCHC, not MCHC concentrate, which may not contain all of the constituents. Some companies have laboratory analyses to confirm that these are indeed all present. No matter how small the amount of each of these substances, it is important that they still be there to maintain the proper proportion of all of the nutrients.

We do know that in secondary osteoporosis MCHC stops the pain which is associated with the frequent fractures. Hairline fractures can be detected throughout the skeletal structure, especially the lower back, in individuals suffering bone loss. Most of the time, individuals just experience the pain without even realizing what is going on. I can tell you, I have seen in my own practice, MCHC reduces and even stops the pain. These effects of MCHC are pretty incredible as all other calcium supplements have proven to have no beneficial effect. Studies have shown that MCHC actually restores lost bone, which cannot be said about any other other calcium or bone supplement.

Some researchers have concluded that the healing process of the fractures commonly seen in osteoporosis victims is aided with the added presence of the matrix crystalline structure. We really don't have all the answers. We just know it seems to be more beneficial than anything we have seen in the past.

Q: MCHC does contain some pretty strange nutrients; platinum, rubidium, silica. Can you elaborate on the importance of these minerals?

Dr. Maher: We know that there are over 60 different minerals in each of our cells in the body. Each of these may have its great importance in making up the entire structure. If some of these are missing, the strength of the entire structure may be weakened. If one just supplements calcium, or calcium and magnesium, which seems to be the consensus of opinion, assuming we absorb them, all these other components are no longer in proportion.

The whole concept is pretty simple. If you have weak bones, "eat" some bone. The nutrients that you need are there.

Q: What dosages of MCHC do you recommend?

Dr. Maher: 1.5 to 3 grams per day depending on the size of the person and the severity of his bone loss. I may recommend up to 10 grams per day in someone with painful fractures.

The best way to treat osteoporosis is with prevention meaning that everyone should examine their individual situation and assess their level of risk. Eliminate as many of the negative behaviors associated with increased risk (smoking, alcohol, coffee and sodas, excess protein, sugar, fat, etc.) as early as possible, exercise regularly, and supplement MCHC in a dosage according to their needs. The sooner in life one practices good bone health, the better they will be in the long run.

Your Osteoporosis Winning Strategy

Osteoporosis is a major public health problem in the United States. The key to its management is prevention by ensuring a balanced diet, adequate amounts of calcium, vitamin D, protein and exercise throughout life. When a significant amount of bone mass has been lost, therapeutic interventions are aimed at preventing further loss with use of antiresorptive agents (ie, estrogen, progestin, calcitonin, and bisphosphonates). Use of pharmacologic agents that stimulate bone formation is still in experimental stages.

Research efforts focusing on prevention, diagnosis, and treatment of osteoporosis are in progress and should provide improved strategies in the future.

1) Bone can be rebuilt. Lost bone can be restored.

2) Supplementing with calcium by itself is not the answer.

This runs counter to two prevailing beliefs. Bone loss, regarded as a more or less unavoidable consequence of aging, is thought to be irreversible. According to the second myth, all we need to do in order to enjoy strong, healthy bones is maintain a high calcium intake, by consuming lots of dairy products, "calcium-fortified" foods and calcium supplements.

Simply increasing calcium intake does not guarantee strong bones. No nutrient functions in isolation. Studies have shown conclusively that neither calcium supplements nor high calcium diets can do much more than slow bone loss down somewhat.

We will all suffer the consequences if we neglect the health of our skeleton. As medical advances continue to insure our chances of living a longer life, the significance greatly is diminished if the quality of those extra years does not improve as well. Life will be sadly wanting if the framework holding us together has deteriorated to the point where we experience constant pain, crippling, and disfigurement, or the inability to engage in normal activities without risking a life-threatening fracture!

We all need to take positive action against bone loss to ensure we do not fall victim to osteoporosis. We need to do this as soon as possible, before bone loss begins. The good news is that if bone loss has already occurred, bone can be restored by taking the proper measures and utilizing supplements such as MCHC. Note the following **Healthy Bone Insurance Factors:**

Avoid eating a diet high in animal protein which induces a calcium deficiency.

Avoid eating sweets and refined carbohydrates which stimulate alkaline digestive juices, making calcium insoluble.

Avoid prolonged stress, alcohol abuse, antibiotics, steroids, and cigarettes.

Make sure you get adequate exercise.

A diet that is adequate in protein, calcium, magnesium, phosphorus, vitamin C, and vitamin D is the best treatment and prevention for osteoporosis.

General healthy bone nutrients:
Vitamin B-12: 30 - 900 mcg daily

Vitamin B-6: 5 - 25 mg daily

Vitamin C: 1,000-2,000 mg 2 to 4 times daily

Vitamin D: 5,000 IU daily

Vitamin E: 600 IU daily

*Calcium: 1 - 2 grams daily

*Magnesium: 500 - 1,000 mg daily

*Copper:

*Phosphorus:

*Silica:

*Boron:

Herbs: Comfrey and Horsetail.

DHEA: Women: 25 mg. one to two times daily

              Men: 25 - 50 mg. one to two times daily

Natural Progesterone

* MCHC provides all of these minerals in a ratio beneficial for absorption and utilization. MCHC, with its highly digestible form of calcium and key calcium synergists, is the only nutritional substance scientifically proven to rebuild lost bone.

Bibliography

Allen SH "Primary osteoporosis. Methods to combat bone loss that accompanies aging." *Postgrad Med* 1993 Jun;93(8):43-6, 49-50, 53-5.

Aloia, J.K., *Metabolism*, 1990: 39: 35-38.

American Journal of Clinical Nutrition, 1982; 35;1048-1075.

Appleton, Nancy, "Healthy Bones" Avery Publishing, Garden City Park, NY,1991.

Benke, P.J. et al, "Osteoporotic bone disease in the pyridoxine deficient rat" *Biochem Med* 1972, 6: 526-535.

Brazier, M., Fardelonne, P., Bollony, R., Sebert, J.L., Desmet,G. *Euro. J. Drug Metab Pharmacokinet* 1991, Spec No 3, pg 161-165.

Brenton, D.P and Dent, C.E. "Ideopathic Juvenile Osteoporosis" *Inborn Errors of Metabolism* Ed. Bickel, H. & Stern J. Publ. MTP Press Limited 1976 pg 222-239.

Chestnut CH 3d "Do we have any alternative to sex steroids in the prevention and treatment of osteoporosis?" *Baillieres Clin Obstet Gynaecol* 1991 Dec;5(4):857-65.

Christianson, D.,et al, *Eur. J. Clin. Invest.* 1981;11: 305-308.

Davies, I.J.T., "Osteogenesis Imperfecta Treated with Microcrystalline Hydroxyapatite Compound" Osteoporosis, A Multi-disciplinary Problem" Ed Dixon. (1983) Royal Society of Medicine International Congress and symposium Series No. 55 Public Academic Press Inc. (London) and Royal Society of Medicine pg, 279-286.

Dawson-Hughes B; Dallal GE; Krall EA; Sadowski L; Sahyoun N; Tannenbaum S A controlled trial of the effect of calcium supplementation on bone density in postmenopausal women. *N Engl J Med* 1990 Sep 27;323(13):878-83.

Dent, C.E., Davies, I.J.T., "Calcium metabolism in bone disease; effects of treatment with microcrystalline calcium hydroxyapatite compound with dihydrotachysterol" Journal of the Royal Society of Medicine, (1980) 73;780-787.

Dodds, R.A. et al "Abnormalities in fracture healing induced by vitamin B-6 deficiency in rats" Bone 1986, 7; 489-495.

Epstein O; Kato Y; Dick R; Sherlock S "Vitamin D, hydroxyapatite, and calcium gluconate in treatment of cortical bone thinning in postmenopausal women with primary biliary cirrhosis." Am J Clin Nutr 1982 Sep;36(3):426-30.

Eriksson SA; Lindgren JU "Combined treatment with calcitonin and 1,25-dihydroxyvitamin D3 for osteoporosis in women." Calcif Tissue Int 1993 Jul; 53(1): 26-8.

Evans, Gary, "There are Two C's in Osteoporosis" Bemidji State University, Bemidji, MN.

Gambacciani M; Spinetti A; Taponeco F; Ciaponi M; Cima GP; Teti GC; Genazzani AR "Prospective evaluation of calcium and estrogen administration on bone mass and metabolism after ovariectomy." *Gynecol Endocrinol* 1995 Jun;9(2):131-5.

Goyer RA; Epstein S; Bhattacharyya M; Korach KS; Pounds J "Environmental risk factors for osteoporosis" *Environ Health Perspect* 1994 Apr;102(4):390-4.

Halpern GM; Van de Water J; Delabroise AM; Keen CL; Gershwin ME "Comparative uptake of calcium from milk and a calcium-rich mineral water in lactose intolerant adults: implications for treatment of osteoporosis." *Am J Prev Med* 1991 Nov-Dec;7(6):379-83.

Hasling C; Charles P; Jensen FT; Mosekilde L "A comparison of the effects of oestrogen/progestogen, high-dose oral calcium, intermittent cyclic etidronate and an ADFR regime on calcium kinetics and bone mass in postmenopausal women with spinal osteoporosis." *Osteoporos Int* 1994 Jul;4(4):191-203.

Hayashi K, Uenoyama K, Matsuguchi N. et al " The affinity of bone to hydroxyapatite and alumina in experimentally induced osteoporosis." *J Arthroplasty* 1989 Sep;4(3):257-62.

Hollo, I., et al., "Osteopenia" *Ann Intern Med,* 1977; 86: 637.

Johnson, C.C., et. al.,"Changes in skeletal tissue during the aging process" *Nutrition Reviews,* 1992;50, no.2, pg 385-387.

Kariya, Y., Watabe S. et al, *J. Biol. Chem* (US) 1990 265 (9);pg5081-5.

Khadzhiev A, Rachev E, Katsarova M, Cherveniashki S "The results of a clinical trial of the preparation Ossopan] *Akush Ginekol* (Sofiia) 1990;29(4):85-7.

Kohara N [Clinical study of concerning factors of decreased bone mineral content in hemodialysis patients] *Nippon Jinzo Gakkai Shi* 1991 Jun;33(6):587-96.

Kveton JF; Friedman CD; Piepmeier JM; Costantino PD "Reconstruction of suboccipital craniectomy defects with hydroxyapatite cement: a preliminary report." *Laryngoscope* 1995 Feb;105(2):156-9.

Landman JO; Schweitzer DH; Frolich M; Hamdy NA; Papapoulos SE "Recovery of serum calcium concentrations following acute hypocalcemia in patients with osteoporosis on long-term oral therapy with the bisphosphonate pamidronate. *J Clin Endocrinol Metab* 1995 Feb;80(2):524-8.

Marsh AG; Sanchez TV; Midkelsen O; Keiser J; Mayor G "Cortical bone density of adult lacto-ovo-vegetarian and omnivorous women." *J Am Diet Assoc* 1980 Feb;76(2):148-51.

Mills, T.J., Davis, H. Broadhurst, B.W. "The Use of Whole Bone in the Treatment of Fracture's" *Manitoba Medical Review*; 1965;45:92-96.

Metz JA; Anderson JJ; Gallagher PN Jr "Intakes of calcium, phosphorus, and protein, and physical-activity level are related to radial bone mass in young adult women" *Am J Clin Nutr* 1993 Oct;58(4):537-42.

Mongiorgi R, Krajewski A "Mineralogical alterations in osteoporotic bone tissue structure." *Biomaterials* 1981 Jul;2(3):147-50.

Nawata H; Tanaka S; Tanaka S; et al "Aromatase in bone cell: association with osteoporosis in postmenopausal women." *J Steroid Biochem Mol Biol* 1995 Jun;53(1-6):165-74.

Neilson, F.H. "Effect of Dietary Boron on Mineral, Estrogen and Testosterone Metabolism in Postmenopausal Women" *FASEB J* 1987;1; 394-297.

Nilsen KH; Jayson MI; Dixon AS "Microcrystalline calcium hydroxyapatite compound in corticosteroid-treated rheumatoid patients: a controlled study." *Br Med J* 1978 Oct 21;2(6145):1124.

Orwoll, E.S., et al "The effects of dietary protein insufficiency and excess on skeletal health" *Bone* 1992; 13;343-350.

Ott, S.M. et al *Ann. Internal Medicine*, 1989;110;267-274.

Parsons, B., Mitchell, C., Emond, A., Darby, A..J., "The Use of Sodium Flouride and Calcium Supplements and Vitamin D in the Treatment of Axial Osteoporosis." "Osteoporosis, A Multi-disciplinary Problem" Ed Dixon. (1983) Royal Society of Medicine International Congress and symposium Series No. 55 Public Academic Press Inc. (London) and Royal Society of Medicine pg, 259-264.

Pfeiffer, Naomi" Moderate Drinking may cut Osteoporosis" *Medical Tribune*, 1992; 3 July23;

Pines A; Raafat H; Lynn AH; Whittington J "Clinical trial of microcrystalline hydroxyapatite compound ('Ossopan') in the prevention of osteoporosis due to corticosteroid therapy." *Curr Med Res Opin* 1984;8(10): 734-42.

Prince R; Devine A; Dick I; Criddle A; Kerr D; Kent N; Price R; Randell A "The effects of calcium supplementation (milk powder or tablets) and exercise on bone density in postmenopausal women. *J Bone Miner Res* 1995 Jul;10(7):1068-75.

Prince RL; Smith M; Dick IM; Price RI; Webb PG; Henderson NK; Harris MM "Prevention of postmenopausal osteoporosis. A comparative study of exercise, calcium supplementation, and hormone-replacement therapy." *N Engl J Med* 1991 Oct 24;325(17):1189-95.

Remagen W; Prezmecky L "Bone augmentation with hydroxyapatite: histological findings in 55 cases." *Implant Dent* 1995 Fall;4(3):182-8.

Reynolds, T.M., "Hip fractures in patients may be vitamin B-6 deficient. Controlled study of serum pyridoxal-5'-phosphate." *Acta Orthop Scand* 1992, 63: 635-638.

Riggs, B.L., et al, " A New Option For Treating Osteoporosis" *New England Journal of Medicine,* (1990) 323:124-125.

Riggs, B.L., et al, " The Prevention and Treatment of Osteoporosis" *New England Journal of Medicine,* 1992;327 (9) 620-627.

Ringe JD, Keller A "Risk of osteoporosis in long-term heparin therapy of thromboembolic diseases in pregnancy: attempted prevention with ossein-hydroxyapatite" *Geburtshilfe Frauenheilkd* 1992 Jul;52(7):426-9.

Roepke, J.B. et al "Effect on smoking and vitamin B-6 supplementation during pregnancy on maternal vitamin B-6 status and infant birth weight" *Fed Proc* 1983, 42:1066.

Rubinacci A; Divieti P; Capponi A; Resmini G; Daverio R; Veglia F; Tessari L "Reduction in parathormone secretion after oral calcium loading in osteoporotic adults" *Endocrinol* 1992 Apr-Jun;17(2):55-65.

Ruegsegger P; Keller A; Dambacher MA "Comparison of the treatment effects of ossein-hydroxyapatite compound and calcium carbonate in osteoporotic females." *Osteoporosis Int* 1995 Jan;5(1):30-4.

Shangraw, R. "Factors to consider in the selection of a calcium supplement" Special Topic Conference on Osteoporosis. October, 1987.

Snow-Harter CM "Bone health and prevention of osteoporosis in active and athletic women." *Clin Sports Med* 1994 Apr;13(2):389-404

Spencer H; Kramer L; Osis D; Wiatrowski E; Norris C; Lender M "Effect of calcium, phosphorus, magnesium, and aluminum on fluoride metabolism in man." *Ann N Y Acad Sci* 1980;355:181-94.

Spencer H; "Effect on small doses of aluminum-containing antacids on calcium and phosphorus metabolism" *American Journal of Clinical Nutrition* 1982; 36:32-40.

Spencer H; Kramer L; et al, "Antacid-induced calcium loss" *Arch Internal Medicine* 1983;143:657-659.

Stamp, T.C.B., Jenkins, M.V. Walker, P.G., and Mitchell, T.H. " Treatment of osteoporosis and MCHC compound and sodium flouride." "Osteoporosis, A Multi-disciplinary Problem" Ed Dixon. (1983) Royal Society of Medicine International Congress and symposium Series No. 55 Public Academic Press Inc. (London) and Royal Society of Medicine pg. 287-290.

Stellon, A., A. Davis., A Webb., and R. Williams. "Microcrystalline Hydroxy apatite compound in prevention of bone loss in corticosteriod-treated patients with chronic actice hepatitis." *Postgraduate Medicine Journal* (1985) 61, 791-796.

Stephan, J.J., Pospichal J., et al. "Prospective Trial of Ossein-Hydroxyapatite compound in surgically induced postmenopausal women." *Bone* (1989) 10, 179-185.

Stevenson JC; Hillard TC; Lees B; Whitcroft SI; Ellerington MC; Whitehead MI "Postmenopausal bone loss: does HRT always work?" Wynn Institute for Metabolic Research, London, U.K. *Int J Fertil Menopausal Stud* 1993;38 Suppl 2:88-91.

Tremollieres F; Pouilles JM; Ribot C "Effect of long-term administration of progestogen on post-menopausal bone loss: result of a two-year, controlled randomized study." *Clin Endocrinol* (Oxf) 1993 Jun;38(6):627-31.

Walker, Alexander "Osteoporosis and Calcium Deficiency" *American Journal of Clinical Nutrition*, Vol. 16, March 1965.

Windsor AC; Misra DP; Loudon JM; Staddon GE "The effect of whole-bone extract on 47 Ca absorption in the elderly." *Age Ageing* 1973 Nov; 2(4): 230-4.

Yamamoto, M.Y., et al *J Clin Invest*, 1984;74: 507-513.

Index

79

BOOKS AVAILABLE FROM BL PUBLICATIONS:

Send book order total amount plus $2 shipping by
check or money order to BL Publications, 21 Donatello,
Aliso Viejo, CA 92656

Health Learning Handbooks

Castor Oil: Its Healing Properties
by Beth Ley   36 pages, $3.95

Dr. John Willard on Catalyst Altered Water
By Beth Ley 60 pages, $3.95

Colostrum: Nature's Gift to the Immune System
By Beth Ley   60 pages, $3.95

**How to Fight Osteoporosis and Win! The Miracle of
Microcrystalline Hydroxyapatite**
By Beth Ley   80 pages, $6.95

The Potato Antioxidant: Alpha Lipoic Acid
By Beth Ley   96 pages, $6.95

Additional Titles

Natural Healing Handbook
by Beth Ley with foreword by Dr. Arnold J. Susser,
R.P., Ph.D. 320 pages, $14.95
(Order by calling toll free: 1-800-507-2665)

How Did We Get So Fat?
By Dr. Arnold J. Susser and Beth Ley, 96 pages, $7.95

A Diet For The Mind By Fred Chapur, 112 pages,
$8.95

**DHEA: Unlocking the Secrets of the Fountain of
Youth** by Beth Ley, 208 pages, $14.95
(Order by calling toll free: 1-800-507-2665)